I0767531

Lymphedema Diet

A Beginner's 4-Step Guide, with Sample Recipes, Meal Plan, and a Food Content Guide

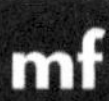

copyright © 2024 Brandon Gilta

All rights reserved No part of this book may be reproduced, or stored in a retrieval system, or transmitted in any form or by any means, electronic, mechanical, photocopying, recording, or otherwise, without express written permission of the publisher.

Disclaimer

By reading this disclaimer, you are accepting the terms of the disclaimer in full. If you disagree with this disclaimer, please do not read the guide.

All of the content within this guide is provided for informational and educational purposes only, and should not be accepted as independent medical or other professional advice. The author is not a doctor, physician, nurse, mental health provider, or registered nutritionist/dietician. Therefore, using and reading this guide does not establish any form of a physician-patient relationship.

Always consult with a physician or another qualified health provider with any issues or questions you might have regarding any sort of medical condition. Do not ever disregard any qualified professional medical advice or delay seeking that advice because of anything you have read in this guide. The information in this guide is not intended to be any sort of medical advice and should not be used in lieu of any medical advice by a licensed and qualified medical professional.

The information in this guide has been compiled from a variety of known sources. However, the author cannot attest to or guarantee the accuracy of each source and thus should not be held liable for any errors or omissions.

You acknowledge that the publisher of this guide will not be held liable for any loss or damage of any kind incurred as a result of this guide or the reliance on any information provided within this guide. You acknowledge and agree that you assume all risk and responsibility for any action you undertake in response to the information in this guide.

Using this guide does not guarantee any particular result (e.g., weight loss or a cure). By reading this guide, you acknowledge that there are no guarantees to any specific outcome or results you can expect.

All product names, diet plans, or names used in this guide are for identification purposes only and are the property of their respective owners. The use of these names does not imply endorsement. All other trademarks cited herein are the property of their respective owners.

Where applicable, this guide is not intended to be a substitute for the original work of this diet plan and is, at most, a supplement to the original work for this diet plan and never a direct substitute. This guide is a personal expression of the facts of that diet plan.

Where applicable, persons shown in the cover images are stock photography models and the publisher has obtained the rights to use the images through license agreements with third-party stock image companies.

Table of Contents

Introduction

Lymphedema, a condition that causes swelling in the body's tissues, is a reality for millions of people worldwide. This often misunderstood and overlooked health concern can significantly impact an individual's quality of life. But there's one key aspect of managing lymphedema that many might not be fully aware of - diet.

The human body functions like a well-oiled machine, with various systems working in unison to maintain our overall health. One such system is the lymphatic system, a network of tissues and organs that help rid the body of toxins and waste. When this system faces disruption, it can lead to lymphedema, a condition that can manifest as discomfort, pain, and mobility issues.

However, hope is not lost. A carefully curated diet can be an effective strategy in managing lymphedema. Imagine a world where you have a better understanding and control over your lymphedema symptoms. That world can become a reality with the right knowledge and tools at your disposal.

Living with lymphedema doesn't mean resigning oneself to a life of discomfort. By gaining insights into the role of diet in lymphedema management, individuals can regain some control over their health. The right dietary choices can help manage symptoms, improve mobility, and enhance the overall quality of life.

In this guide, we will talk about the following;

- What Is Lymphedema?
- Stages of Lymphedema
- What are The Symptoms of Lymphedema?
- How Is Lymphedema Diagnosed?
- How is lymphedema treated?
- The Lymphedema Diet
- Principles, Benefits, and Disadvantages of Lymphedema Diet
- A Step-by-step Guide to Get Started with the Lymphedema Diet
- Foods to Eat and To Avoid
- Sample Meal Plan and Recipes

Are you prepared to unlock the potential of diet in managing lymphedema? Let's commence this journey of exploration as we delve into the scientific aspects of lymphedema and the significant influence of diet on its management. This guide is poised to offer practical advice and invaluable information to assist you in making lymphedema-friendly dietary choices.

Through this guide, you'll gain more than just knowledge about lymphedema; you'll acquire a toolset to help manage the condition more effectively. Let's embark on this journey towards better understanding and management of lymphedema today.

Chapter 1: What Is Lymphedema?

Lymphedema is a condition characterized by the accumulation of fatty tissue deposits under the skin. It acts as a blockage in the lymphatic system, causing swelling of some body parts and immediate discomfort. This swelling is usually observed in one's legs or arms, but may also occur in the neck, face, belly, trunk, and even the genitals. Clinically, it has two types: primary lymphedema and secondary lymphedema.

Stages of Lymphedema

Lymphedema is commonly classified into four stages, each representing a different level of severity:

- **Stage 0 (Latent or Subclinical)**: In this stage, there may not be noticeable changes in the size or shape of the affected limb or area, but lymphatic transport is already impaired. The patient might experience a sensation of heaviness, tightness, or fullness in the limb, but no visible swelling is present. This stage can last for months or even years before progressing.
- **Stage 1 (Mild)**: At this stage, the limb or body part begins to swell and feels heavier. The swelling is often soft, and pressing on the skin will leave an indentation, a condition known as pitting edema. The good news is that this stage is reversible; elevating the limb often reduces the swelling, and proper treatment can return the limb to its normal size.

- **Stage 2 (Moderate)**: In this stage, the affected limb becomes increasingly swollen. The tissue starts to feel firmer and pitting may be less obvious or absent. The skin may start to take on a spongy consistency and begin to harden, a condition known as fibrosis. This stage of lymphedema is not reversible with elevation, but it can still be managed with appropriate treatment.
- **Stage 3 (Severe)**: Also known as lymphostatic elephantiasis, this is the most advanced stage of lymphedema. The swelling is extreme, and the affected limb or body part may become very large. The skin is hard and thickened and may develop folds, crevices, or warty overgrowths. This stage can be challenging to manage and may significantly impact the patient's mobility and quality of life.

These stages help doctors determine the best treatment plan for each individual. It's important to note that progression through these stages is not inevitable, especially with early diagnosis and appropriate management.

What are The Symptoms of Lymphedema?

Lymphedema is a chronic disease that can manifest through various symptoms. It's important to note that these symptoms can range from mild to severe, and they may develop gradually over time. Here are some common signs and symptoms of lymphedema:

- **Swelling**: This is the most common symptom of lymphedema. It usually affects an arm or a leg, but it can also occur in other parts of the body. The swelling is due to a buildup of lymph fluid, which can't be properly drained because of damage to the lymphatic system.

- **Feeling of heaviness or tightness**: Individuals with lymphedema often report a sensation of heaviness or tightness in the affected limb. This feeling is due to the increased volume of fluid in that area.
- **Restricted range of motion**: Due to the swelling and discomfort, people with lymphedema may have difficulty moving the affected limb freely. This can interfere with daily activities and overall quality of life.
- **Aching or discomfort**: Lymphedema can cause aching, discomfort, or even pain in the affected area. This discomfort can vary in intensity and may worsen throughout the day.
- **Recurring infections**: Because the lymphatic system plays a crucial role in the immune response, damage to this system can lead to an increased risk of infections, particularly skin infections.
- **Hardening and thickening of the skin (fibrosis)**: Over time, the ongoing inflammation and swelling can cause changes in the texture of the skin. It can become hard, and thick, and may take on a lumpy appearance.

Remember, if you suspect you have lymphedema or are experiencing any of these symptoms, it's crucial to seek medical advice. Early diagnosis and treatment can help manage the symptoms and prevent the progression of the condition.

What are the causes of lymphedema?

Lymphedema is typically caused by damage to or removal of lymph nodes, leading to a blockage in the lymphatic system. This blockage prevents lymph fluid from draining well, and as the fluid accumulates, the swelling characteristic of lymphedema occurs.

There are two types of lymphedema, each with distinct causes:

Primary Lymphedema

This is a relatively rare condition that is often inherited. It arises from anomalies in the formation and development of the lymphatic system, specifically the lymph vessels. These are crucial for the body's immune response and fluid balance, so any irregularities can cause issues such as lymphedema.

Primary lymphedema can manifest at any stage of life, but it's commonly observed to start during infancy, adolescence, or early adulthood.

The specific timing often depends on the subtype of primary lymphedema, which is categorized based on its onset:

Congenital Lymphedema

This subtype is present from birth or makes its appearance shortly thereafter. Infants with congenital lymphedema may exhibit noticeable swelling in one or both limbs due to the accumulation of lymph fluid.

This condition results from genetic mutations that affect the formation of the lymphatic system. Despite its early onset, with appropriate management, children with congenital lymphedema can lead healthy and active lives.

Lymphedema Praecox (Meige's Disease)

This is the most common form of primary lymphedema, typically developing during the period of puberty, although it can appear anytime before the age of 35. The onset often coincides with hormonal changes, growth spurts, or physical trauma.

The swelling can affect any part of the body, but it frequently impacts the lower extremities. Symptoms may include a feeling of heaviness, discomfort, or recurrent infections in the affected area.

Lymphedema Tarda

This subtype usually begins after the age of 35, hence the term 'tarda' meaning late. It's less common than lymphedema praecox, but it shares many of the same symptoms, including swelling in one or more parts of the body, feelings of tightness or fullness, and recurring infections. The late onset can sometimes lead to a delay in diagnosis, making it all the more important for adults to seek medical attention if they notice persistent swelling.

Each subtype of primary lymphedema requires its own specific management and treatment strategy, which may include physical therapy, compression garments, or surgery in some cases. Early detection and intervention are key to managing the symptoms and preventing the progression of the condition.

Secondary Lymphedema

This form of lymphedema is more prevalent than primary lymphedema. It's not due to an inherited or congenital defect but instead is caused by damage to the lymphatic system.

Various factors can contribute to this damage:

Cancer Treatments

Secondary lymphedema is most frequently associated with treatments for cancer that involve the removal of or damage to lymph nodes or lymph vessels. For instance, in the management of breast cancer, it may be necessary to remove lymph nodes from the armpit area to prevent the spread of the disease.

This surgical procedure can disrupt the normal flow and drainage of lymph fluid, leading to accumulation and subsequent swelling characteristic of lymphedema. Not everyone who has such surgery will develop lymphedema, but the risk is present and increases with the number of lymph nodes removed.

Infections

Certain infections, particularly those caused by parasites, can lead to secondary lymphedema. Filariasis, a parasitic infection spread by mosquitoes in tropical and subtropical regions, is a common cause. The parasites invade the lymphatic system, causing inflammation and damage which leads to impaired lymph drainage and subsequently lymphedema.

Injury or Trauma

Traumatic injuries, including burns, wounds, or other physical traumas, can damage the lymphatic system and result in lymphedema. This could occur as a result of an accident, severe skin infection, or even certain types of surgery unrelated to cancer treatment.

Radiation Therapy

Radiation therapy, another common treatment for various types of cancers, can also lead to secondary lymphedema. High-energy radiation can cause scarring and inflammation of the lymphatic system. This can impair the ability of the lymph vessels to effectively transport lymph fluid, leading to its accumulation and consequent swelling.

Secondary lymphedema can be a challenging condition to manage due to its association with other serious health issues like cancer. However, with careful monitoring, early detection, and appropriate treatment, including physical therapy, compression devices, medications, and sometimes surgery, it is possible to manage the symptoms and prevent further complications.

It's important for patients undergoing treatments or procedures that could affect the lymphatic system to be aware of the signs of lymphedema and to seek medical advice promptly if they notice any changes.

How Is Lymphedema Diagnosed?

Diagnosing lymphedema is a multi-step process that involves a thorough evaluation of the patient's medical history and symptoms, followed by a physical examination and possibly some diagnostic tests. Here is a more detailed look into each step:

1. **Medical History**: The healthcare provider will begin by collecting a detailed medical history. This includes asking about any past surgeries, radiation treatments, or other medical procedures that might have caused damage to the lymphatic system. The provider may also ask about any recurring infections or symptoms such as persistent swelling.

2. **Physical Examination**: Following the discussion of the patient's medical history, a physical examination is conducted. The healthcare provider will visually inspect for signs of swelling and skin changes in the affected area. In addition, the provider may measure the circumference of the affected limb at different points to assess the degree of swelling.

3. **Imaging Tests**: Depending on the findings from the medical history and physical examination, the healthcare provider may order imaging tests to further investigate. These could include:

- **Lymphoscintigraphy**: A test that uses a small amount of radioactive material to highlight the lymphatic system in images.
  - **MRI or CT Scans**: These scans provide detailed images of the body's tissues and structures, helping to rule out other potential causes of swelling.
  - **Doppler Ultrasound**: An ultrasound that evaluates blood flow in the vessels and can help rule out venous disease, which can also cause swelling.
4. **Bioimpedance Analysis (BIA)**: This is a newer technique that measures the amount of fluid in the body's tissues. It involves passing a small electrical current through the body and measuring the resistance to this current. This test can be particularly useful in the early detection of lymphedema.
5. **Indocyanine Green Lymphography (ICG)**: This is another imaging technique that uses a fluorescent dye to visualize the lymphatic vessels. The dye is injected into the body and then illuminated with a special light, allowing physicians to observe how the dye moves through the lymphatic system.

It's important to note that the diagnosis of lymphedema can be complex and may require multiple tests and evaluations. If you notice persistent swelling or other potential signs of lymphedema, it's crucial to seek medical advice promptly.

Lifestyle Changes to Manage Lymphedema

Managing lymphedema often involves making key lifestyle changes to help control symptoms and prevent the condition from worsening. Here are some common recommendations:

- **Exercise**: Regular, gentle exercise can help promote lymph drainage. Activities like walking, swimming, yoga, and stretching can be beneficial. Always consult with your healthcare provider or a physical therapist before starting any new exercise regimen.
- **Healthy Diet**: Maintaining a healthy weight through a balanced diet can reduce strain on the lymphatic system. It's also important to stay hydrated, but avoid alcohol and salty foods as these can encourage fluid retention and swelling.
- **Skin Care**: Good skincare routines are essential to prevent infections, which can worsen lymphedema. This includes keeping skin clean and moisturized, avoiding cuts and burns, and treating any wounds promptly.
- **Compression Garments**: Wearing specially designed compression garments can help prevent fluid build-up and promote the flow of lymph. These should be worn as recommended by your healthcare provider.
- **Elevation**: Elevating the affected limb above the level of your heart when possible can help encourage lymph flow.
- **Avoid Tight Clothing**: Tight clothes, jewelry, or watches can restrict lymph flow. Wear loose clothing and avoid anything that could constrict the affected area.

- **Avoid Heat**: Exposure to high heat can cause fluid accumulation, so it's best to avoid hot baths, saunas, and sunbathing.
- **Avoid Heavy Lifting**: Lifting heavy objects can put a strain on the lymphatic system. If you need to lift something, be sure to use proper form and avoid straining the affected limb.
- **No Blood Pressure Readings or Injections**: Avoid having blood pressure readings taken or receiving injections in the affected arm to prevent further damage to the lymphatic system.

These lifestyle changes can significantly help in managing lymphedema symptoms and improving quality of life. It's always best to consult with a healthcare provider for personalized advice and treatment plans.

How is lymphedema treated?

The treatment for lymphedema varies depending on the stage of the condition and the severity of the symptoms. Here's a more organized version of the information provided:

Lymphedema can be categorized into three stages: Stage 1 (Spontaneous Lymphedema), Stage 2 (Spontaneous Irreversible), and Stage 3 (Lymphostatic Elephantiasis). The treatment approach differs for each stage.

In Stage 1, the condition is still reversible as the soft tissue under the skin remains undamaged. While treatment at this stage doesn't guarantee the prevention of future lymphedema, many individuals who receive appropriate treatment at this stage do not experience further issues. However, it's important to note that there's still a risk for the disease to progress to a more severe stage.

For later stages of lymphedema, the treatment options depend on the severity of the symptoms and how well the patient's body responds to the treatment. Individuals with mild symptoms that only occasionally worsen may only need regular, consistent treatment.

However, those with persistent or severe symptoms might require more active, ongoing treatment. It's also worth mentioning that lymphedema tends to have a dynamic nature, meaning symptoms can fluctuate over time.

Non-surgical treatments are typically recommended for early-stage lymphedema. These may include medication, manual compressions, and dietary adjustments. In more advanced stages, surgical intervention may be necessary to remove excess tissue and fluid.

Manual compressions can take several forms, including:

- **Stockings or Elastic Sleeves**: These provide graduated compression from the extremities towards the trunk, promoting lymph flow.
- **Bandages**: Wrapped tightly around the extremities and looser at the trunk, these assist in directing lymph flow toward the body's center.
- **Pneumatic Compression Devices**: These are pump-connected stockings or sleeves that provide sequential compressions, aiding lymph flow from the

extremities to the trunk. They're often used at home or in clinics and can help prevent long-term scarring. However, they're not suitable for patients with deep venous thrombosis, certain infections, or heart failure.

- **Manual Lymph Drainage**: This massage technique manually compresses the muscles to stimulate lymph flow.

In conclusion, while the treatment for lymphedema varies, it often involves a combination of dietary changes, manual compressions, and potentially surgery in more severe cases.

Chapter 2: The Lymphedema Diet

We have already discussed some of the treatments made if you are diagnosed with lymphedema. One of these treatments is to undergo the "Lymphedema Diet". This diet aims to include foods that will not worsen the swelling of the lymph, thus, alleviating other symptoms too.

In general, it is advised to watch out for salty foods because the sodium in them increases the retention of fluid in the body. Moreover, with the increased fluid retention because of excessive salt intake, blood pressure will also increase, making lymphedema symptoms worse.

Principles of The Lymphedema Diet

The principles of the Lymphedema Diet, as suggested by various sources, revolve around promoting healthy lymphatic function and alleviating symptoms. Here are some key principles:

- **Balanced Nutrition**: A diet rich in fruits, vegetables, lean proteins, healthy fats, and whole grains is recommended.
- **Limit Sodium**: High sodium intake can lead to fluid retention, so it's advised to limit salt intake.
- **Adequate Protein**: Protein is essential for repairing tissues and maintaining a strong immune system, hence its importance in the diet.

- **Avoid Alcohol, Caffeine, and Diuretics**: These substances can dehydrate the body and exacerbate swelling.
- **Healthy Weight Management**: Maintaining a healthy weight can help alleviate symptoms and prevent additional strain on the lymphatic system.
- **Hydration**: Keeping hydrated is crucial, but avoid alcohol and caffeinated drinks as they can lead to dehydration.
- **Consideration of Dietary Approaches**: Some sources suggest that specific dietary approaches, like a ketogenic diet, may help reduce lymphatic swelling. However, this should always be discussed with a healthcare provider.
- **Overall Lifestyle Management**: Alongside diet, managing stress, getting enough sleep, and regular exercise are also important.

Remember, individual needs can vary, so it's always best to consult with a healthcare provider or a registered dietitian to personalize dietary plans and strategies.

Benefits of Lymphedema Diet

Incorporating the principles of a lymphedema diet into your lifestyle can provide numerous benefits, including:

- **Reduced Swelling**: By limiting sodium, which can cause fluid retention, you can help reduce swelling in affected limbs.
- **Enhanced Immune Function**: A diet rich in fruits, vegetables, and lean proteins provides essential

nutrients that can boost the immune system and help the body fight off infections.

- **Weight Management**: Maintaining a healthy weight can lessen the strain on the lymphatic system, helping to control lymphedema symptoms.
- **Improved Overall Health**: A balanced, nutritious diet supports overall health, reducing the risk of other health problems like heart disease, diabetes, and certain cancers.
- **Increased Energy Levels**: Good nutrition can improve energy levels, making it easier to stay active and manage symptoms.
- **Improved Skin Health**: Adequate hydration and essential nutrients help maintain skin health, which is crucial in preventing infections that could worsen lymphedema.
- **Better Fluid Balance**: Proper hydration helps maintain the body's fluid balance, aiding in the management of lymphedema.

Remember, individual results may vary, and it's important to consult with a healthcare provider before making significant dietary changes.

Disadvantages of The Lymphedema Diet

Though the benefits of a lymphedema diet generally outweigh the disadvantages, it's important to acknowledge potential challenges:

- **Dietary Restrictions**: The need to limit certain foods, like those high in sodium or processed items, may feel restrictive and could lead to feelings of deprivation.
- **Time and Effort**: Preparing fresh, whole foods can be time-consuming. It may also require learning new cooking techniques or recipes.
- **Cost**: Fresh, organic produce and lean proteins can be more expensive than processed foods, which may impact the budget.
- **Initial Adjustment Period**: Changing dietary habits can be challenging at first and may cause temporary digestive discomfort as your body adjusts.
- **Limited Immediate Results**: Improvements in lymphedema symptoms may not be immediately noticeable, which can be discouraging for some people.

Despite these challenges, the long-term health benefits of a lymphedema diet, such as reduced swelling, enhanced immune function, improved overall health, and better fluid balance, make it a valuable part of managing this condition. As always, any dietary changes should be discussed with a healthcare provider to ensure they're suitable for individual needs.

Chapter 3: A step-by-step Guide To Getting Started with The Lymphedema Diet

To help you get started, it is important to follow these four general steps to head start your way to the lymphedema diet:

Step 1: Limit your sodium intake

The human body requires a balance of water and salt, also known as sodium, for proper physiological function. However, consuming an excessive amount of salty foods can disrupt this balance and lead to health complications.

Sodium plays a major role in regulating the volume of fluid that is in or around cells, including blood cells. When we consume a high-sodium diet, our bodies retain more water to dilute the sodium. This excess water increases the volume of blood flowing through vessels, which in turn raises the pressure on arterial walls - a condition known as high blood pressure.

High blood pressure can lead to the filtering out of more substances by the blood capillaries, which can further contribute to the swelling of the lymph, a condition known as lymphedema. Lymphedema is characterized by swelling in your arms or legs due to a blockage in your lymphatic system, which prevents lymph fluid from draining well.

In addition to the potential for causing fluid imbalance, foods high in sodium are often heavily processed and therefore tend to contain fewer nutrients. These foods may not provide the necessary vitamins and minerals that your body needs to function optimally.

Some common examples of high-sodium foods include cheese, bread, salad dressings, sauces, shellfish, deli meats, canned foods, and pizza. These foods are often a staple in many diets, so it's essential to be mindful of portion sizes and consider healthier alternatives when possible.

To manage sodium intake, consider cooking at home more often, where you can control the amount of salt added to your meals. Also, try incorporating more fresh fruits and vegetables into your diet, as these are naturally low in sodium. Lastly, make a habit of reading food labels to choose lower-sodium options.

Limiting sodium intake is a crucial step in managing lymphedema and maintaining overall health. Always consult with a healthcare provider or dietitian for personalized advice on dietary changes.

Step 2: Level up your protein intake

Protein plays a vital role in our bodies, performing various functions such as repairing body tissues, making hormones and enzymes, aiding in the growth and development process, and acting as essential building blocks for bones, muscles, cartilage, skin, and blood.

One of the key proteins found in our bodies is albumin, which is also a significant component of lymph fluid. The lymphatic system, part of our immune system, relies on this protein-rich fluid to function optimally. Albumin helps maintain the right balance of fluid in your body by drawing excess fluid from tissues back into the bloodstream.

Contrary to what some might think, reducing protein intake does not necessarily lead to a decrease in lymph fluid. In fact, adequate protein intake is crucial in replacing the proteins lost along with the lymph fluid. This is especially important in managing conditions like lymphedema, where the lymphatic system's normal functioning is compromised, leading to protein-rich fluid build-up in body tissues.

Protein can be obtained from various dietary sources. Examples include low-fat cheese, lean chicken, fish, tofu, low-fat veal, and lean beef. These protein sources are not only rich in essential amino acids but they also contribute to a balanced diet that supports overall health.

It's important to note that protein needs can vary depending on several factors. For instance, if you're dealing with muscle wasting, engaging in increased physical activities, undergoing medical treatment, healing wounds or sores, or as you age, your protein requirements may be higher.

In these cases, it's crucial to adjust your protein intake accordingly to ensure your body gets the necessary nutrients for repair and recovery. Always consult with a healthcare provider or dietitian to determine the appropriate amount of protein for your specific circumstances.

In conclusion, leveling up your protein intake is a significant step in managing lymphedema and supporting overall bodily functions. It's not just about consuming more protein, but ensuring you're getting the right amount from quality sources.

Step 3: Drink water, not alcohol

Hydration is a fundamental aspect of maintaining overall health and wellness. While there may not be a direct correlation between fluid retention and fluid intake, drinking an adequate amount of fluids, particularly water, is crucial for numerous bodily functions.

Water plays a pivotal role in our bodies, acting as a medium for various chemical reactions. It aids in the removal of waste and toxins through excretion, helps maintain body temperature, supports digestion, transports nutrients, and even lubricates joints. These functions are critical for overall health and also directly or indirectly support the functioning of the lymphatic system.

The National Cancer Institute recommends consuming 8 to 12 glasses of water per day, although the exact amount can vary based on factors such as age, sex, weight, activity level, and overall health. Keeping yourself adequately hydrated can help ensure your body functions optimally and could potentially aid in managing conditions like lymphedema.

On the other hand, alcohol is a substance that should be limited, especially if you have lymphedema. Alcohol can lead to dehydration, which can exacerbate symptoms of lymphedema. It can also impair the immune system, which relies on the lymphatic system to function effectively. Moreover, alcohol has diuretic properties, meaning it can increase urine production and potentially lead to further fluid imbalance.

Alcohol can also contribute to weight gain, another factor that can worsen lymphedema symptoms. Excess body weight puts additional pressure on already compromised lymph vessels, making it harder for them to move lymph fluid effectively.

In conclusion, prioritizing hydration and limiting alcohol consumption are vital aspects of managing lymphedema and supporting overall health. Always remember to consult with a healthcare provider or dietitian for personalized advice on fluid intake and alcohol consumption.

Step 4: Choose your dietary fats

The types of fats you consume can significantly impact your health, particularly if you're managing a condition like lymphedema. One of the primary functions of the lymphatic system is to absorb dietary fats and transport them to the bloodstream. However, not all fats are absorbed and transported in the same way.

Medium Chain Triglycerides (MCTs) are a type of fat that behaves differently from most other fats in our diet. Unlike long-chain fatty acids, which require the lymphatic system for absorption and transportation, MCTs are absorbed directly into the bloodstream through the gut. This process bypasses the lymphatic system, thus reducing its workload.

Research suggests that incorporating more MCTs into your diet could potentially decrease the likelihood of experiencing symptoms of lymphedema. By easing the burden on the lymphatic system, these fats could help manage and prevent further swelling associated with this condition.

Sources of MCTs include palm oil and coconut oil. These oils can be used in cooking or baking as a substitute for other types of fats. Another common source of MCTs is dairy products, although the concentration is significantly lower than in oils.

However, it's important to remember that while MCTs can be beneficial, they are still a form of saturated fat. Consuming too much-saturated fat can increase your risk of heart disease and other health conditions. Therefore, it's crucial to balance your intake of MCTs with other healthy fats such as monounsaturated and polyunsaturated fats found in foods like avocados, nuts, seeds, and fatty fish.

As always, when making dietary changes, it's essential to consult with a healthcare provider or dietitian to ensure you're meeting your nutritional needs and managing your health conditions effectively.

In conclusion, being selective about the types of fats you consume can play an essential role in managing lymphedema. Opting for fats like MCTs that reduce the workload on the lymphatic system could potentially help manage this condition while supporting overall health.

Food Content Guide for Lymphedema

You already know how to spot what you can eat and what you cannot. To help you more in this journey, here are three lists that will talk about food you can eat, what you can eat (but not always), and food you should rarely or NEVER eat.

List 1: What should you always eat?

These are foods that are generally fine to consume as long as they are still within the recommended intake. Up to half a cup of some of these are fine to consume. Just always remember that there is no good in eating too few and too much. Everything should be in the right amount.

- Adzuki beans
- Amaranth
- Apples
- Apricots
- Bananas
- Beans
- Beets
- Black beans
- Blackberries
- Blueberries
- Brown rice
- Buckwheat
- Butter beans
- Cannellini beans
- Cherries
- Chickpeas
- Coffee
- Corn

- Cranberries
- Dark, green, and leafy vegetables
- Fava beans
- Fermented foods
- Frozen or fresh berries
- Garlic
- Grapefruit
- Grapes
- Great northern beans
- Herbs
- Kidney beans
- Kiwi fruit
- Legumes
- Lentils
- Lima beans
- Mangoes
- Melons
- Milk
- Millet
- Mushrooms
- Navy beans
- Oatmeal
- Onions
- Oranges
- Papaya
- Peaches
- Pears
- Peas
- Peppers
- Pineapple
- Pinto beans

- Plums
- Pulses
- Quinoa
- Raspberries
- Red, purple potatoes
- Sorghum
- Squash
- Strawberries
- Sweet potatoes
- Tea
- Teff
- Unsweetened cocoa
- Wild rice
- Yams

List 2: What you should eat in limited quantities

These are foods that you can eat but with some discretion. You can consume around 6-8 servings of the foods here per week. They are on the "limited" list because they contain food components that may worsen the lymphedema symptoms if eaten in normal amounts.

- Brazil nuts
- Butter
- Dark chocolate
- Dried fruits
- Duck
- Fish rich in omega-3 fatty acids like wild salmon, mackerel, tuna, herring, anchovies, and sardines
- Free-range meat

- Get sugar from fruits
- Ghee
- Goat cheese
- Milk
- Organic chicken without skin
- Organic Dairy
- Organic eggs
- Red wine
- Sheep cheese
- Turkey
- Unprocessed cheese
- Unsalted and raw seeds and nuts
- Unsaturated fats

List 3: What you should rarely or never eat?

If some of the foods here are your favorites, unfortunately, you can only eat them rarely or even never. You can eat these if you are feeling special or have something to celebrate. But be a mindful eater and make sure that you remember them being on this list.

- Alcohol
- Backed products
- Chips
- Crisps
- Fries
- Grain products with gluten
- Pasta
- Pizza
- Processed meat

- Saturated fats
- Soy
- Sweet drink
- Sweet foods

Chapter 4: Sample 7-Day Meal Plan

So, you are now very familiar with what you can consume. This chapter will help you formulate your meals. To keep you started, here is a 7-day meal plan based on the foods that you can eat.

Most of the foods that you are allowed to eat are generally healthy whole foods. So, you can mix them up to make your meals and create variations to what is available to you. As a bonus, some of the recipes for the dishes stated in the meal plan are shown in the last part. Feel free to use them in your diet!

Sunday

Breakfast

- Whole grain toast with almond butter and banana slices

Lunch

- Turkey and Avocado Wrap on Whole-Grain Tortilla, side of baby carrots

Dinner

- Grilled Chicken Breast with Steamed Asparagus and Wild Rice

Monday

Breakfast

- Greek yogurt with mixed berries and a sprinkle of granola

Lunch

- Spinach and Feta Salad with a light vinaigrette

Dinner

- Baked Salmon with a lemon dill sauce, a side of quinoa, and green beans

Tuesday

Breakfast

- Scrambled eggs with sautéed bell peppers and onions

Lunch

- Tuna Salad on whole-grain bread, side of cucumber slices

Dinner

- Lemon Herb Roasted Turkey Breast with steamed broccoli and sweet potato mash

Wednesday

Breakfast

- Smoothie made with spinach, pineapple, and coconut water

Lunch

- Chickpea and Vegetable Soup with a slice of whole-grain bread

Dinner

- Grilled Shrimp Skewers with brown rice and mixed vegetables

Thursday

Breakfast

- Oatmeal topped with fresh fruit and a drizzle of honey

Lunch

- Chicken Caesar Salad (use low-sodium dressing)

Dinner

- Baked Cod with a tomato and basil sauce, side of couscous and asparagus

Friday

Breakfast

- Whole grain pancakes with blueberries and a dollop of Greek yogurt

Lunch

- Quinoa and Black Bean Salad with a lime vinaigrette

Dinner

- Roasted Pork Tenderloin with a side of mashed cauliflower and steamed green beans

Saturday

Breakfast

- Chia seed pudding made with almond milk and topped with mixed berries

Lunch

- Vegetable Stir Fry with tofu served over brown rice

Dinner

- Grilled Steak with a side of baked sweet potato and steamed zucchini

Remember to also drink plenty of water throughout the day, aiming for 8-12 glasses. Always consult with a healthcare provider or dietitian before making significant changes to your diet. This meal plan is a suggestion and may need to be adjusted based on individual dietary needs and preferences.

Chapter 5: Sample Recipes

Following are some sample recipes that incorporate the tips mentioned in this guide. Remember, these recipes are just a starting point and you can always modify them to suit your personal taste and dietary restrictions.

Grilled Shrimp Skewers with Brown Rice and Mixed Vegetables

Ingredients:

For the Grilled Shrimp Skewers:

- 1 pound large shrimp, peeled and deveined
- 2 tablespoons olive oil
- 2 cloves garlic, minced
- Zest and juice of 1 lemon
- Salt and pepper to taste
- 8 skewers (if using wooden skewers, soak them in water for 20 minutes prior to grilling)

For the Brown Rice:

- 1 cup brown rice
- 2 cups water or low-sodium vegetable broth

For the Mixed Vegetables:

- 4 cups mixed vegetables of your choice (e.g., bell peppers, broccoli, carrots, zucchini)
- 1 tablespoon olive oil
- Salt and pepper to taste

Instructions:

1. **Get the shrimp ready:** Take a bowl and mix with the shrimp, minced garlic, lemon juice, lemon zest, olive oil, salt, and pepper. Ensure that the shrimp are thoroughly coated by tossing them in the mixture. Proceed to arrange the shrimp on the skewers.

2. **Cook the brown rice:** Rinse the rice under cold water until the water runs clear. In a pot, bring the water or broth to a boil. Add the rice, reduce heat to low, cover, and simmer for about 45 minutes, or until the rice is tender and all the liquid is absorbed.

3. **Grill the shrimp skewers:** Preheat your grill or grill pan over medium-high heat. Grill the shrimp skewers for 2-3 minutes on each side, or until the shrimp are pink and cooked through.

4. **Saute the vegetables:** While the shrimp are grilling, heat the olive oil in a large pan over medium heat. Add the mixed vegetables, season with salt and pepper, and sauté until the vegetables are tender-crisp, about 5-7 minutes.

5. **Serve:** Divide the cooked brown rice among four plates. Top each with a serving of sautéed vegetables and two shrimp skewers.

Scrambled Eggs with Spinach

Ingredients:

- 4 large eggs
- 1 cup fresh spinach leaves
- 1 tablespoon of coconut oil
- Salt and pepper to taste

Instructions:

1. Crack the eggs into a bowl and whisk them until the yolks and whites are fully combined. Season with a pinch of salt and pepper.
2. Heat the coconut oil in a non-stick frying pan over medium heat.
3. Add the fresh spinach leaves to the pan. Cook for 2-3 minutes, or until the spinach has wilted.
4. Pour the beaten eggs over the wilted spinach. Let the eggs cook for a minute, or until they start to set around the edges.
5. Stir the eggs and spinach gently with a spatula, pushing it from one side of the pan to the other. Continue to cook for another minute or until the eggs are cooked to your liking.
6. Once done, remove the pan from the heat. You can add a sprinkle of extra black pepper on top if you like.
7. Serve hot with a piece of whole-grain toast if desired.

Grilled Chicken Salad

Ingredients:

For the salad:

- 2 boneless, skinless chicken breasts
- 4 cups mixed salad greens
- 1 cup cherry tomatoes, halved
- 1 cucumber, sliced

For the dressing:

- 3 tablespoons extra-virgin olive oil
- 1 tablespoon lemon juice
- Salt and pepper to taste

Instructions:

1. Season the chicken breasts with salt and pepper. Grill over medium-high heat for 5-7 minutes on each side, or until the internal temperature reaches 165°F (74°C). Let the chicken rest for a few minutes before slicing it into thin strips.
2. While the chicken is grilling, prepare your salad base. In a large bowl, combine the mixed salad greens, cherry tomatoes, and cucumber slices.
3. To make the dressing, whisk together the extra-virgin olive oil and lemon juice in a small bowl. Season with salt and pepper to taste.
4. Once the chicken is cooked and sliced, add it to the salad bowl.

5. Drizzle the olive oil dressing over the salad and toss gently to combine, ensuring all ingredients are lightly coated in the dressing.

6. Serve immediately, or refrigerate until ready to eat.

Baked Salmon with Steamed Broccoli and Quinoa

Ingredients:

- 2 salmon filets
- 1 tablespoon of olive oil
- Salt and pepper to taste
- 1 lemon, sliced
- 2 cups of fresh broccoli florets
- 1 cup of quinoa
- 2 cups of water or low-sodium vegetable broth

Instructions:

1. Preheat your oven to 400°F (200°C). Line a baking sheet with foil for easy cleanup.
2. Place the salmon filets on the baking sheet. Drizzle with olive oil and season with salt and pepper. Top each filet with a couple of lemon slices.
3. Bake in the preheated oven for 12-15 minutes, or until the salmon is cooked through and flakes easily with a fork.
4. While the salmon is baking, prepare the quinoa. Rinse the quinoa under cold water until the water runs clear. This helps to remove any bitterness.
5. Add the rinsed quinoa and water or broth to a saucepan. Bring to a boil, then reduce heat to low, cover, and let it simmer for about 15 minutes, or until the quinoa has absorbed all the liquid. Let it sit off the heat for 5 minutes, then fluff with a fork.

6. Steam the broccoli florets until they are tender-crisp, about 5 minutes. You can do this in a steamer or the microwave with a little bit of water.

7. Serve each salmon filet with a side of steamed broccoli and a scoop of quinoa.

Tofu Stir-Fry

Ingredients:

- 1 block of firm tofu, drained and cubed
- 2 tablespoons of coconut oil
- 2 cloves of garlic, minced
- 1 red bell pepper, sliced
- 1 yellow bell pepper, sliced
- 2 cups of broccoli florets
- 1 carrot, peeled and sliced into thin rounds
- 2 tablespoons of low-sodium soy sauce or tamari
- 1 tablespoon of sesame oil
- Salt and pepper to taste

Instructions:

1. Press the tofu to remove excess moisture. To do this, wrap the tofu in a clean kitchen towel or paper towel, place it on a flat surface, and put a heavy object on top (like a pan or a cutting board). Leave it for about 15-20 minutes.
2. Once the tofu is pressed, cut it into cubes.
3. Heat the coconut oil in a large wok or frying pan over medium-high heat.
4. Add the tofu cubes to the pan and cook until they are golden brown on all sides, about 5-7 minutes. Remove the tofu from the pan and set it aside.
5. In the same pan, add the minced garlic, sliced bell peppers, broccoli florets, and carrot rounds. Stir-fry the vegetables for about 5 minutes, or until they are tender-crisp.

6. Return the tofu to the pan with the vegetables. Add the low-sodium soy sauce or tamari and sesame oil. Stir everything together and cook for another 2-3 minutes.
7. Season with salt and pepper to taste.
8. Serve hot, preferably with a side of brown rice or quinoa if desired.

Grilled Lean Beef Steak with Sweet Potato and Mixed Vegetables

Ingredients:

- 2 lean beef steaks
- Salt and pepper to taste
- 2 medium sweet potatoes
- 1 tablespoon olive oil
- 2 cups mixed vegetables (such as bell peppers, zucchini, and carrots), chopped
- 1 garlic clove, minced

Instructions:

1. Preheat your grill to medium-high heat.
2. Season the beef steaks with salt and pepper. Grill them for 4-6 minutes per side, or until they reach your desired level of doneness. Let the steaks rest for a few minutes before serving.
3. While the steaks are grilling, prepare your sweet potatoes. Wash and scrub the sweet potatoes, then cut them into cubes. Toss the cubes in olive oil, then spread them out on a baking sheet.
4. Roast the sweet potato cubes in a preheated oven at 400°F (200°C) for about 20 minutes, or until they are tender and slightly caramelized.
5. To prepare the mixed vegetables, heat a bit of olive oil in a pan over medium heat. Add the minced garlic and cook until fragrant, about 1 minute.

6. Add the chopped vegetables to the pan and sauté until they are tender-crisp, about 5-7 minutes. Season with salt and pepper to taste.

7. Serve each grilled steak with a side of roasted sweet potatoes and sautéed mixed vegetables.

Baked Cod

Ingredients:

- 2 cod filets
- Salt and pepper to taste
- 1 lemon, sliced
- 2 cups of green beans, ends trimmed
- 2 cloves of garlic, minced
- 1 tablespoon of olive oil
- 1 cup of couscous
- 2 cups of water or low-sodium vegetable broth

Instructions:

1. Preheat your oven to 400°F (200°C). Line a baking sheet with foil for easy cleanup.
2. Place the cod filets on the baking sheet. Season with salt and pepper and top each filet with a couple of lemon slices.
3. Bake in the preheated oven for 12-15 minutes, or until the cod is cooked through and flakes easily with a fork.
4. While the cod is baking, prepare the green beans. Heat the olive oil in a pan over medium heat. Add the minced garlic and cook until fragrant, about 1 minute.
5. Add the green beans to the pan and sauté until they are tender-crisp, about 5-7 minutes. Season with salt and pepper to taste.
6. To prepare the couscous, bring the water or broth to a boil in a saucepan. Stir in the couscous, then remove from heat, cover, and let sit for 5 minutes. Fluff with a fork before serving.

7. Serve each baked cod filet with a side of garlic green
    beans and a scoop of couscous.

53

Turkey and Avocado Wrap

Ingredients:

- 2 whole-grain tortillas
- 4 slices of low-sodium turkey breast
- 1 ripe avocado, sliced
- Lettuce leaves
- 1 medium tomato, sliced
- Salt and pepper to taste
- 1 cup of baby carrots

Instructions:

1. Lay out the whole-grain tortillas on a clean surface.
2. Arrange 2 slices of turkey breast on each tortilla.
3. Add lettuce leaves and tomato slices on top of the turkey.
4. Peel and slice the avocado, then add the slices to the tortillas.
5. Season with a little bit of salt and pepper to taste.
6. Roll up the tortillas tightly, then cut each wrap in half.
7. Serve each wrap with a side of baby carrots.

Grilled Chicken Breast with Steamed Asparagus and Wild Rice

Ingredients:

- 2 boneless, skinless chicken breasts
- Salt and pepper to taste
- 1 bunch of fresh asparagus, ends trimmed
- 1 cup of wild rice
- 2 cups of water or low-sodium chicken broth

Instructions:

1. Preheat your grill to medium-high heat.
2. Season the chicken breasts with salt and pepper. Grill them for 6-8 minutes per side, or until they reach an internal temperature of 165°F (74°C). Let the chicken rest for a few minutes before serving.
3. While the chicken is grilling, prepare the asparagus. Place the asparagus in a steamer basket over a pot of boiling water. Cover and steam for about 3-5 minutes, or until the asparagus is tender-crisp. Season with a bit of salt and pepper to taste.
4. To prepare the wild rice, bring the water or broth to a boil in a saucepan. Stir in the rice, then reduce the heat to low, cover, and let simmer for about 45 minutes, or until the rice is tender and has absorbed all the liquid.
5. Serve each grilled chicken breast with a side of steamed asparagus and a scoop of wild rice.

Spinach and Feta Salad

Ingredients:

For the Salad:

- 4 cups of fresh spinach leaves
- 1 cup of cherry tomatoes, halved
- 1 cucumber, sliced
- 1/2 red onion, thinly sliced
- 1/2 cup of crumbled feta cheese

For the Vinaigrette:

- 1/4 cup of extra virgin olive oil
- 2 tablespoons of apple cider vinegar
- 1 teaspoon of Dijon mustard
- 1 garlic clove, minced
- Salt and pepper to taste

Instructions:

1. In a large bowl, combine the spinach leaves, cherry tomatoes, cucumber slices, and red onion.
2. To prepare the vinaigrette, whisk together the olive oil, apple cider vinegar, Dijon mustard, and minced garlic in a small bowl. Season with salt and pepper to taste.
3. Drizzle the vinaigrette over the salad and toss gently to combine.
4. Sprinkle the crumbled feta cheese on top of the salad just before serving.

Lemon Herb Roasted Turkey Breast with Steamed Broccoli and Sweet Potato Mash

Ingredients:

For the Turkey:

- 1 boneless turkey breast (about 2-3 pounds)
- 2 cloves garlic, minced
- Zest and juice of 1 lemon
- 2 tablespoons olive oil
- 1 teaspoon dried rosemary
- 1 teaspoon dried thyme
- Salt and pepper to taste

For the Broccoli:

- 1 large head of broccoli, cut into florets
- Salt to taste

For the Sweet Potato Mash:

- 2 large sweet potatoes, peeled and cubed
- 1 tablespoon olive oil
- Salt and pepper to taste

Instructions:

1. **For the Turkey:** Preheat your oven to 375°F (190°C). In a small bowl, combine the minced garlic, lemon zest, lemon juice, olive oil, rosemary, thyme, salt, and pepper. Rub this mixture all over the turkey breast.

2. Place the turkey breast in a roasting pan and roast for about 60-75 minutes, or until the internal temperature reaches 165°F (74°C). Once cooked, let the turkey rest for 10 minutes before slicing.

3. **For the Broccoli:** While the turkey is roasting, steam the broccoli florets until they are bright green and tender-crisp, about 5 minutes. Season with a little salt.

4. **For the Sweet Potato Mash:** Boil the sweet potato cubes until they are soft, about 15-20 minutes. Drain well, then mash with the olive oil until smooth. Season with salt and pepper.

5. Serve the sliced turkey with steamed broccoli and sweet potato mash on the side.

Chia Seed Pudding with Almond Milk and Mixed Berries

Ingredients:

For the Chia Seed Pudding:

- 1/4 cup of chia seeds
- 1 cup of unsweetened almond milk
- 1 tablespoon of honey or maple syrup (optional)

For the Topping:

- 1/2 cup of mixed berries (such as blueberries, raspberries, and strawberries)

Instructions:

1. In a bowl or mason jar, combine the chia seeds and unsweetened almond milk. Stir until well combined.
2. If you like your pudding a bit sweet, add a tablespoon of honey or maple syrup and stir again.
3. Cover the mixture and refrigerate for at least 4 hours, or overnight.
4. Once the chia seeds have absorbed the almond milk and the mixture has thickened into a pudding-like texture, give it a good stir.
5. Top the chia seed pudding with a generous serving of mixed berries.
6. Enjoy your chia seed pudding immediately, or cover and refrigerate to enjoy later!

Tuna Salad on Whole-Grain Bread with a side of Cucumber Slices

Ingredients:

For the Tuna Salad:

- 1 can of low-sodium tuna in water, drained
- 2 tablespoons of low-fat Greek yogurt
- 1 tablespoon of Dijon mustard
- 1/4 cup of finely chopped celery
- 1/4 cup of finely chopped red onion
- 1/4 teaspoon of black pepper
- A pinch of sea salt (optional)

For the Sandwich and Side:

- 2 slices of whole-grain bread
- A handful of fresh lettuce leaves
- 1 medium cucumber, sliced

Instructions:

1. In a bowl, combine the drained tuna, Greek yogurt, Dijon mustard, celery, red onion, black pepper, and a pinch of sea salt (if using). Mix until well combined.
2. Lay out the two slices of whole-grain bread. Spread the tuna salad evenly over one slice.
3. Top the tuna salad with fresh lettuce leaves, then place the second slice of bread on top to complete the sandwich.
4. Serve the sandwich with a side of fresh cucumber slices.

Roasted Pork Tenderloin with Mashed Cauliflower and Steamed Green Beans

Ingredients:

For the Roasted Pork Tenderloin:

- 1 pound pork tenderloin
- 1 tablespoon olive oil
- A pinch of black pepper
- A pinch of sea salt (optional)
- 1 teaspoon dried thyme
- 1 teaspoon dried rosemary

For the Mashed Cauliflower:

- 1 head of cauliflower, cut into florets
- 1/4 cup unsweetened almond milk
- 1 tablespoon olive oil
- A pinch of black pepper
- A pinch of sea salt (optional)

For the Steamed Green Beans:

- 2 cups fresh green beans, ends trimmed
- A pinch of black pepper
- A pinch of sea salt (optional)

Instructions:

1. Preheat your oven to 400°F (200°C). Rub the pork tenderloin with olive oil, then season with black pepper, sea salt (if using), thyme, and rosemary. Place

on a baking tray and roast in the oven for about 20-25 minutes, or until the internal temperature reaches 145°F (63°C).

2. While the pork is roasting, steam the cauliflower florets until they are very soft. Once cooked, drain and transfer to a food processor. Add the almond milk, olive oil, black pepper, and sea salt (if using). Process until smooth and creamy.

3. Steam the green beans until they are just tender. Season with a pinch of black pepper and sea salt (if using).

4. Once the pork is cooked, remove it from the oven and let it rest for a few minutes before slicing.

5. Serve the sliced pork tenderloin with a side of mashed cauliflower and steamed green beans.

Chicken Caesar Salad with Low-Sodium Dressing

Ingredients:

For the Chicken Caesar Salad:

- 2 boneless, skinless chicken breasts
- 1 tablespoon olive oil
- A pinch of black pepper
- A pinch of sea salt (optional)
- 6 cups romaine lettuce, chopped
- 1/4 cup grated Parmesan cheese

For the Low-Sodium Caesar Dressing:

- 1/2 cup Greek yogurt
- 1 clove garlic, minced
- 1 tablespoon lemon juice
- 1 tablespoon olive oil
- 1 teaspoon Dijon mustard
- A pinch of black pepper
- A pinch of sea salt (optional)

Instructions:

1. Preheat your grill or stove-top grill pan over medium heat. Rub the chicken breasts with olive oil, then season with black pepper and sea salt (if using).
2. Grill the chicken for about 5-7 minutes on each side, or until the internal temperature reaches 165°F (74°C). Once cooked, let it rest for a few minutes before slicing.

3. As the chicken takes a breather, get started on the low-sodium Caesar dressing. Take a bowl and mix in it the Greek yogurt, olive oil, minced garlic, Dijon mustard, lemon juice, black pepper, and sea salt (if you're using any). Stir the mixture thoroughly until it's well blended.

4. In a large salad bowl, toss the chopped romaine lettuce with the prepared Caesar dressing until well coated. Top the dressed lettuce with the sliced grilled chicken and sprinkle with grated Parmesan cheese.

5. Serve the Chicken Caesar Salad immediately.

How to Sustain this Diet

You are already aware of the general rules, of what to eat and what not to eat, and you have an idea of how you can plan your meals. In this chapter, you will be given tips on how to sustain the diet, as well as be successful in it. Here are the tips:

Know your alternatives

The lymphedema diet is not that strict compared to other diets. It only needs to watch out mostly for salty, processed, and overly sweet foods. So, it is important to know what you can replace with a certain food item that you want.

For example, if you are fond of eggs, you can still eat them. But be mindful of how you can still improve this choice. In this case, instead of eating eggs from strict poultry farms, you can opt for organic eggs because these are more natural, less processed, and contain more nutrients.

Cook your meals

Most fast foods, food stalls, and even restaurants use a tremendous amount of salt in their foods because salt makes food much more savory. So, to skip overthinking whether you consume excess salt whenever you eat out, learn how to cook your meals.

At least, this makes you learn a helpful survival skill. At the same time, you get to choose the meals, the ingredients, and how you would prepare them. It is the perfect time for experimentation.

Replace salt with herbs

It cannot be denied that most delicious and flavorful foods contain a lot of salt in them. But remember the first tip? Know your alternatives! Instead of salt, why not try herbs and spices? These are valid ingredients that give a boost of flavor, too.

Besides, they provide therapeutic and healing effects in the body. Using herbs and spices is also an exploration because combining them creates a new dimension of flavor that even salt alone cannot give.

Exercise

Of course, to help with your lymphedema, an exercise that involves the stimulation and contraction of muscles is important because this helps the lymph work. Exercise, in general, also helps you stay alive, alert, and awake. So it is not only the symptoms of your lymphedema being cured, but your life for sure will lean more toward wellness if you exercise regularly.

Be a mindful eater

Know what you eat. This is important because the consumption of items that are not ideal for your condition may bear consequences that might come off worse than what you are currently feeling. This tip also involves not starving yourself as you will start to binge eat if you are hungry.

And when you are binge eating, you do not care about how much food you eat, and if it is good or not good for you. Be responsible and disciplined enough to know your boundaries as someone with lymphedema.

Conclusion

Congratulations! You've made it to the end of this comprehensive guide on the lymphedema diet. We're genuinely proud of you for taking this crucial step towards understanding and managing your condition. This journey has been about more than just learning; it's about taking charge of your health and making informed decisions that positively affect your life.

Throughout this guide, you've gained an in-depth understanding of what lymphedema is, how it affects your body, and most importantly, how specific dietary choices can help manage its symptoms. You've discovered that it's not just about what you eat, but also when and how you eat it. By now, you should feel empowered, and armed with the knowledge necessary to navigate your way through managing this condition.

Remember, the key to a successful lymphedema management strategy lies in maintaining a balanced diet—plenty of fruits, vegetables, lean proteins, and whole grains. Hydration is equally important, so ensure you're drinking enough water throughout the day. But remember, it's not just about what you eat, but also about maintaining a healthy lifestyle overall. Regular exercise, stress management, and proper sleep are all critical components of managing lymphedema effectively.

It's essential to remind yourself that every individual is unique. What works well for one person might not work as well for another. So, while this guide provides a general roadmap, customizing these recommendations to fit your personal needs, preferences, and lifestyle is crucial. Don't be afraid to experiment with different foods and recipes, always keeping in mind the guiding principles we've discussed.

Living with lymphedema can indeed pose challenges, but remember, you're not alone in this journey. Many have walked this path before you and have successfully managed their symptoms through dietary changes and lifestyle modifications. You too can do it!

In conclusion, we hope this guide has served as a valuable resource for you. The knowledge you've gained will hopefully inspire you to make positive dietary changes and lead a healthier life. Remember, managing lymphedema is a journey, not a destination. It's about making small, sustainable changes that add up over time.

Thank you for spending your time with us, for investing in your health, and for choosing to educate yourself. We wish you all the best on your journey towards better health. Here's to taking control of your lymphedema and living your best life!

Remember, you've already taken the most significant step - starting. Keep going, stay positive, and believe in your ability to make the changes necessary for a healthier future. You've got this!

FAQs

What is a lymphedema diet?

A lymphedema diet is a dietary plan designed to help manage and alleviate the symptoms of lymphedema. It emphasizes consuming anti-inflammatory foods, staying well-hydrated, and maintaining a healthy weight.

Are there specific foods I should avoid with lymphedema?

Yes, it's recommended to limit your intake of processed foods, high-sodium foods, and alcohol as these can exacerbate lymphedema symptoms by causing fluid retention.

What types of foods are beneficial for lymphedema?

Foods rich in antioxidants and anti-inflammatory properties such as fruits, vegetables, lean proteins, and whole grains are beneficial for lymphedema. They can help reduce inflammation and support overall lymphatic function.

Can diet alone cure lymphedema?

No, while a healthy diet can significantly help manage lymphedema symptoms and improve your quality of life, it cannot cure the condition. Lymphedema management typically involves a combination of treatments including physical therapy, compression garments, and sometimes surgery, along with dietary changes.

How does hydration impact lymphedema?

Staying well-hydrated is vital for lymphedema management. Adequate hydration helps maintain the body's fluid balance, supports immune function, and aids in the proper functioning of the lymphatic system.

Is it necessary to lose weight if I have lymphedema?

Maintaining a healthy weight can help manage lymphedema symptoms. Obesity can put additional strain on the lymphatic system, so if you're overweight, losing weight might help alleviate your symptoms. Always consult with a healthcare professional before starting any weight loss program.

Can I still enjoy my favorite foods with lymphedema?

Yes, the lymphedema diet is about balance and moderation. While it's important to focus on nutritious, anti-inflammatory foods, you can still enjoy your favorite treats in moderation. It's about making informed choices that support your overall health and lymphedema management.

References and Helpful Links

Atopic dermatitis (eczema) - Symptoms and causes - Mayo Clinic. (2023, May 9). Mayo Clinic. https://www.mayoclinic.org/diseases-conditions/atopic-derma titis-eczema/symptoms-causes/syc-20353273

Carter, J. (2020, May 26). *Lymphedema & Nutrition - Melanie Massey Physical Therapy*. Melanie Massey Physical Therapy. https://mmptinc.com/lymphedema-nutrition/

Holmes, R. (2021, May 25). *What's involved in a lymphedema diet?* LIVESTRONG.COM. https://www.livestrong.com/article/193714-diet-for-lymphede ma/

DiSipio, T., Rye, S., Newman, B., & Hayes, S. C. (2013). Incidence of unilateral arm lymphoedema after breast cancer: a systematic review and meta-analysis. *The Lancet Oncology*, *14*(6), 500–515. https://doi.org/10.1016/s1470-2045(13)70076-7

National Organization for Rare Disorders. (2023, November 20). *Filariasis - symptoms, causes, treatment | NORD*. https://rarediseases.org/rare-diseases/filariasis/

Foods that may help with swelling and lymphedema. (2024, February 7). This Is Living With Cancer | Official Site. https://www.thisislivingwithcancer.com/content/foods-that-m ay-help-with-swelling-and-lymphedema/

Grada, A., & Phillips, T. J. (2017). Lymphedema. *Journal of the American Academy of Dermatology*, *77*(6), 1009–1020. https://doi.org/10.1016/j.jaad.2017.03.022

MacGill, M. (2024, January 22). *What does the lymphatic system do?* https://www.medicalnewstoday.com/articles/303087

Duncan Gumaer. (2018, August 16). *Lymphedema diet and exercise therapy*. Griswold Home Care. https://www.griswoldhomecare.com/blog/2018/august/lymph edema-diet-and-exercise-therapy/

StÖPpler, M. C., MD. (2023, December 14). *Lymphedema Treatment, Causes, Symptoms, therapy, stages*. MedicineNet. https://www.medicinenet.com/lymphedema/article.htm

Lymphedema - Symptoms and causes - Mayo Clinic. (2022, November 24). Mayo Clinic. https://www.mayoclinic.org/diseases-conditions/lymphedema/ symptoms-causes/syc-20374682

Riches, P. (2019, April 9). *What is lymphedema?* https://www.medicalnewstoday.com/articles/180919

Douketis, J. D. (2024, January 25). *Overview of the lymphatic system*. MSD Manual Consumer Version. https://www.msdmanuals.com/home/heart-and-blood-vessel-d isorders/lymphatic-disorders/overview-of-the-lymphatic-syste m

Rheumatoid arthritis | CDC. (n.d.). https://www.cdc.gov/arthritis/types/rheumatoid-arthritis.html

Sleigh, B. C. (2023, April 19). *Lymphedema*. StatPearls - NCBI Bookshelf. https://www.ncbi.nlm.nih.gov/books/NBK537239/

Admin. (2021, October 18). *What foods should you avoid if you have lymphedema?* Caring Touch Medical. https://www.caringtouchmed.com/what-foods-should-you-avoid-if-you-have-lymphedema/

What is lymphedema? | American Cancer Society. (n.d.). American Cancer Society. https://www.cancer.org/cancer/managing-cancer/side-effects/swelling/lymphedema/what-is-lymphedema.html

www.ingramcontent.com/pod-product-compliance
Lightning Source LLC
Chambersburg PA
CBHW050848260726
48660CB00006B/2508